# NUMBER NINE

*Girly Fears of a Confident Women*

**Saina**

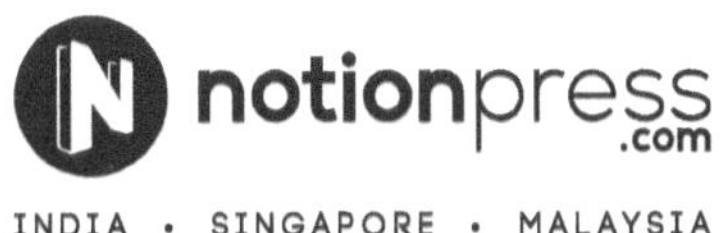

INDIA • SINGAPORE • MALAYSIA

# Notion Press

No.8, 3rd Cross Street,
CIT Colony, Mylapore,
Chennai, Tamil Nadu – 600004

First Published by Notion Press 2021
Copyright © Chirashree Behura 2021
All Rights Reserved.

ISBN 978-1-63832-567-3

## Disclaimer:

This book is based on the experience of a mom who shares her journey towards motherhood, her fears, and her approach to gain back the confidence that she lost in the path. She modifies her life events and shares the tips that enabled her to take good care of her health and the baby's, however, every pregnancy is different and so is every child. Please ensure that you talk to your health care professionals and consultants before accepting/taking any health-based decisions.

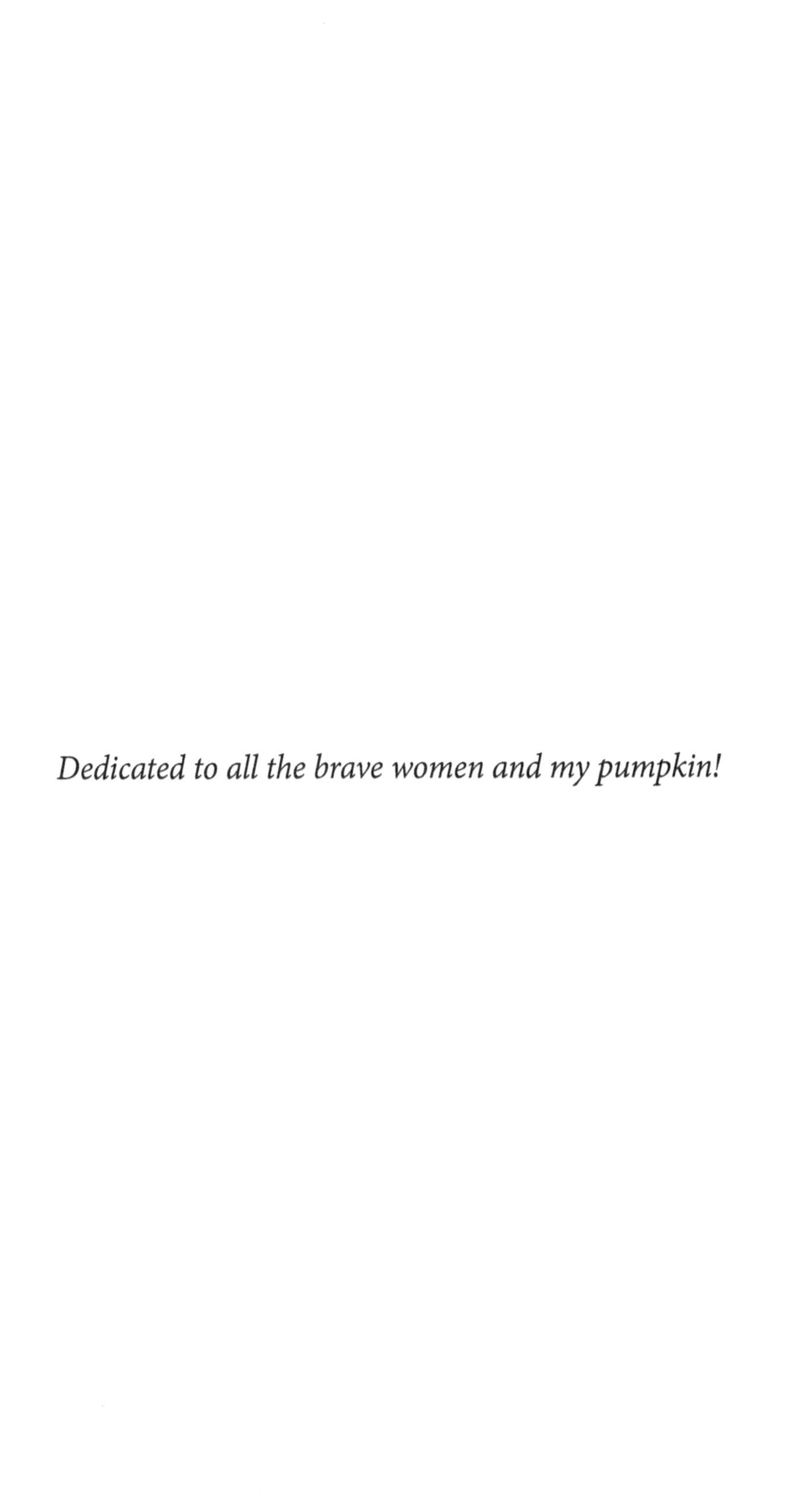

*Dedicated to all the brave women and my pumpkin!*

# Contents

## Impatient World



## Loosing Selfhood



## Plums and Pumpkins



## A New Life – the Unbounded Discovery

# Introduction

'Number Nine' is the reflection of a woman whose fears and confidence are real. A girl with a not-so-easy childhood, a successful working professional fortunate enough to have a wonderful husband, feared pregnancy and its after-effects. She loved kids but feared the dark tunnel that could stall her career, take away her achievements and put her back in the place where she started from. She had other secret fears that she had to overcome to get into the phase of motherhood and gain the wisdom of relationship and reality. The girly thoughts, the fear, the happiness, newborn care, new mom's trouble, and a new world of discovery. Anin shares her experience as a new mom, her postpartum issues, her learnings through pregnancy, the ways of beating the depression and anxiety that comes with the new never-ending responsibility, and the importance of taking the right decisions as per the priorities. This book has all of it; sweet, silly and the girly!

Being a girl, have you ever come across a casual funny remark where you were termed as complicated, confused, unsure and unwilling? I came across it a multiple times and was bold enough to laugh at it. But honestly, who is not? Every human being at some point of time is confused, complicated in an unwanted situation, and unsure when forced to do things unwillingly. I believe that the lucky ones get it less and the brave ones often!

Although it can happen at all phases of life; for we women, its mandated all-at-once when we get married. Expectations, responsibilities, work, insecurities and more. Priorities shuffle and play merry-go-round and we try to hold them all. By the time we settle down and breathe, it will be a new life surrounded by uncertainties and insecurities. It is obvious to get confused, to have secret fears and weird thoughts, but it is important to bounce back and talk to trusted people who could enable us to take the right decision. Anin, as a mom went through all of it, shares her experiences with other women and wish them luck. Stay less confused, have less fear and be brave to take the decision based on your preferences and wishes.

A toast to women!

# Perception and the Fear

# Typical Day at Office

Petrichor was in the air; the weather was pleasant, and a group of girls awaiting hot coffee at the basement of the office were giggling at girly chitchats. The coffee seller swiftly handed over the paper cups to all. Anin and Tracy were in a haste to finish the last drop before throwing the disposable cups in the bin. Tracy's inquisitiveness about Anin's personal life has always been troublesome so Anin deviated her attention towards the conference and veered towards the lift. Tracy followed her; however, she was not one of those who gets distracted easily.

"Hey! You still did not answer about your family plans. Are you trying to ignore me? You know the clock is ticking!", Tracy said while crossing the security desk.

"O Tracy! I have ample of time for that. It is just three years of marriage. Let me do something with this life before I declare myself old and wise", Anin answered.

Tracy dialed in, and as quick as birds, they were all ears at the conference. Tracy acknowledged Rob's queries on the upcoming project delivery dates in affirmative while Anin struggled to stay calm. Anin has always respected personal spaces, even with the best of her friends. With Tracy, she has always been skeptical.

It was very cold in the evening. Anin finished her work and left office around 8:00 PM, dropped Tracy on her way back home and parked the car at the 'corn corner' near her apartment. She treated herself with the famous spinach and corn wrap to feel better but was still not able to let her thoughts go; she was constantly thinking about her colleagues and their secret intentions. Anin always considered herself too young for the family planning stuff. Tired of her restless mind, she reached home. She heard Aakish's footsteps. Oh yes! she can identify it even in crowded places. She kept the door open for him and was all smiling.

They make a great couple together. I can listen to their sweet conversations all day long without getting bored. I feel that they are made for each other; they talk alike, think alike, and welcome each other's opinion and decision effortlessly. They truly share their life!

They watched the continuation episode from the thriller series and shared their days experience. Aakish has always been the matured one and has been expressive about his thoughts. He advised Anin to ignore small things, especially the discussions at office.

"Career, promotions and good twists are all in our cards and we have a lot before planning for the baby. We both must focus on our career and plan for a better world for ourselves. May be after a few years, we can think about the generation ahead", he said crisp and loud unaware of the relief he bestowed on Anin with the answer.

His answer alleviated Anin's restlessness. They enjoyed their pasta with potato wedges; one of their dinner favorites and discussed about their dream home. Their new house was ready, and the plan was to get it registered soon.

More than the calculations and financial planning, it was the interiors that Anin was worried about and Aakish laughed it loud.

# The Curious World

Delighted with their first dream home, the couple hosted a small party. Decors with yellow, not so popular theme for the housewarming ceremony was finalized. Anin later confessed that the color theme was the priest decision as per their tradition, however, it was a crowning achievement for her, a big hit!

Yellow lilies were the wonders of the day. Anin bought a yellow gown for herself and looked pretty in her gorgeous dress; her hairs tied with handmade lilies, the sparkling heels, and her contagious smile, all adding up to her beauty. Believe me, she is still busy collecting the compliments!

Aakish was Anin's only family; Aakish's few cousins were remarkably close to him and were helping him with his new home arrangements. As per the rituals, the offerings were made, and the family enjoyed a get-together. Anin's friends and colleagues had an amazing time at the party with the music and dancing options around. Photo shoot was the catch of the day. Aakish's friends enjoyed the 'self-make ice-cream corner'. Everyone was overjoyed at the glance of the marvelous cake and loved the feast, except for the one concern they all had in common. They all wanted to know if there are any special announcements, but there was none.

It was getting dark, so the guests thanked the couple for the wonderful time and bid goodbye. What astonished me was the sweet and fancy ways in which people reiterated the fact that it is time for the couple to consider the family name retention.

They made it clear; with the completion of five years of marriage and with a new house, "The Spring is over"!

Anin was not happy with the advices offered as she wanted to collect her compliments, think about her new house and nothing else.

"Well organized buffet, dance floors and more; was it not enough for the guests?", asked Anin.

"Well, it is just the human nature. The society we live in is more inclined towards the belief of having a baby within three years of marriage. They get skeptical about the bonding and the wellbeing of the couple when they take a decision to hold any more than the "defined usual""; Aakish said while signing off the final cheque to the vendor.

As always, they discussed the topic in length. They too wanted a small world, a small family; however, they wanted to flourish and have securities in place before taking up responsibilities as parents. Aakish was expecting a promotion at workplace and Anin was doing well as a management trainee so they parked the advices aside and continued with their new home delights. Saturday nights were lively; Sunday was for movies and eat-outs, and weekdays were going well.

# Secret Fears

Having an early morning coffee with Anin was very dear to me. Sharing of our deepest secrets were often initiated with our coffee chats. Soul friends since childhood, we used to read each other's mind and face at times! Anin looked confused and worried so I initiated the conversation, and she told me the reasons of her being skeptical about family planning. It might not be a concern for all, however, majority of women struggling between household and office work agree about the secret fears associated with the pregnancy.

In her own words, she elucidated.

**Fear 1:**

I fear additional responsibilities. With Aakish's free-go-lucky attitude, am spending all my leisure's doing household chores. With all this and a full-time job at office, embracing mom's job is scary and am not ready. I think I can never be!

**Fear 2:**

Shh! Am secretly scared of losing my freedom and everything else. My career is sure to halt for a while. All that I have achieved over the years will vanish. I have worked hard in the past and I love to look back and feel proud of working those extra hours with dedication. Having a baby early can scatter my career plans. Late nights would no longer be on my cards. We might not get the "our time" after long tiring weekdays. I see some of my colleagues skipping day trips because of kids at home. I too realize that the ladies do their best to honor their work and do not hesitate to work extra, however, some people at office do not understand the kind of dedication they show towards their work. I cannot even imagine getting into that situation. Yes, am concerned.

**Fear 3:**

And my looks! What if Zumba or Aerobics cannot help me get back in shape? I know myself; I will never be able to devote time towards reshaping my body. Will I really have time for grooming? What if Aakish stay happy for a while and then get disinterested in me? God forbid but what if this happens! He is my only family. What if I become the lady who gains weight after her pregnancy and never reverts to the same jolly bubbly girl because of the additional responsibilities that pour in? Am not sure if I will be able to handle it.

**Fear 4:**

Let us assume that all goes well and god bestows me with some superpowers. Am still not ready to accept the word "mom" and "the responsibilities associated with it". I can get fascinated with baby's smile, the small feet, but will I be able to take up the onus that is associated with the bundle of joy? Cute and innocent; the baby deserves more caring and responsible mom than I believe I can ever become.

Sighs.

"So, is that all?", I asked.

Yeah, she answered.

"People say that my brain never shuts; I overthink. I understand that free mind is the key, but my overthinking has never harmed me, except for some sleepless nights that I can afford", she added.

We had a long conversation, and I was convinced that she needs more time to get into parenting. It is fair to take additional time when you are not ready. It is equally important to think about the situation before planning unless your biological clock is ticking and you are willing to go ahead with the big decision.

# Convincing Selfhood

# Focused Mindset Alteration

The work pressure at office was tremendous for Anin. She was terribly upset with her unmanaged schedules, her daily chores, and her little puppy.

"It is time to take control of my own life. I should focus on my family. We should first settle down and then start following our dreams rather than just going with the flow and being a part of the race", she said.

Whatever you say sweetheart; answered Aakish.

It was raining and Aakish was cleaning his vibrant collection of flowerpots. I was staring at the lamp post; the flickering light was improvising the raindrops, making it more prominent. The drops were dense, but my eyesight was strong enough to penetrate through them. I saw a lady sitting and smiling near the window of her apartment. She made her cat comfortable in a basket and left in haste. It was difficult for me to track her, but I was trying to see through. She stopped at the shop in the end of the lane. Wind was strong; her scarf almost flew away, however, she had firm hands. She struggled to close her umbrella when the shopkeeper handed over a packet. I got distracted and spilled the coffee.

Anin wanted to talk to me alone so we went inside.

"I observed that all my friends and acquaintances had trouble adjusting at an early stage. They sacrificed something or the other, they got frustrated at a point, complained about their life and family not being supportive; however, no one ever regretted having a baby of their own. What do you think?", she asked.

"That's right! Baby's smiles make the days more cheerful and fulfilling. Maybe the baby helped them forget their worries and sacrifices. Being with the baby never approves of a sad pause. The little being can change a life completely and can make you see only the positive side at times", I answered.

"But is that a good enough reason to have a baby? Is it not worth dedicating your life doing good? Maybe educating a few unprivileged kids. Maybe cleaning some streets where villagers pass by. Educating the girls at the farm about the personal hygiene. Will that not make us smile? Will that not make us happy?", asked Anin.

"Why not? Doing good is a blessing. It is a practice and is no way related to the baby. Having a baby or not, is a personal choice and should not be mixed with other feelings. The little one will not stop you from doing what you want to. Doing good deeds with the baby might help you contribute more towards the society. We not just serve but also act as role models for the next generations, the foundation of giving and caring. The choice is yours! I have seen people completely devoting their life serving others and earning a good night sleep", I answered with a smile.

Yeah, that is right; answered Anin.

The conversation she had with me that day was different. She was slowly preparing herself for the next phase of her life, which was a good sign considering the couples priority.

# Confident Pre-Pregnancy Checks

Anin was aware of the rewards associated with the pre-pregnancy checks. Pre-pregnancy consultations not just help us gain insight but also make us aware of any hidden health issues that we might have with respect to pregnancy. Common issues like thyroids, etc. can effortlessly be controlled these days with the medicines prescribed by the doctor prior to pregnancy planning. Regular checkups, doctor visits, timely medicines and proper scanning hold the power to make a women confident and enable them to enjoy the pregnancy bliss.

With each passing day, Anin's feeling of a "would-be graceful mom" was getting stronger. The best of her friend becoming a mother of a cute baby girl was encouraging and she was slowly preparing herself to walk on the same lane. She was also preparing Aakish thoughtfully for the big step.

One day while coming back from office she visited a clinic, paid the consultation fees, and waited for her turn at the lobby. Nervous when Aakish called her, she did not disclose her whereabouts. When the nurse gestured her to go inside the doctor's room, she was nervous and excited at the same time.

"How can I help?", the doctor asked.

She sounded like a teacher to her and Anin was prepared to be her obedient student.

"Am thirty-two (32) years old and never pregnant. I feel it's time to plan for my pregnancy, so is there anything that I must know?", Anin asked.

"Well, there are a few tests that we can go for but before that you need to give me some information about yourself and your family", the doctor said.

"I would like to know if you have any family history of thyroid, disabilities, genetic disorders that you are aware of"; the doctor asked.

"No disabilities for sure, but I don't know much. All I could say that I have no issues as such", Anin answered.

"Ok, No worries. We have ways to find out. I will prescribe few tests which is usually done to ensure that your body is ready for the pregnancy. First test is to ensure about the vaccinations that you would have taken against some viral infections, second is for thyroid and the third is a routine blood checkup. If these three shows well, we are good to go", the doctor said.

Anin kept the prescription in her laptop holder and was happy to know that there were no physical examinations. She was one of those ladies who believed that checkups related to pregnancy can be scary and messy. Next day, she woke up early, secretly went to the nearby lab and gave the blood sample for testing. She then came home and geared up for her office. Just then Aakish woke up and found Anin rushing towards the door.

"Do you have an early morning meet by any chance?", Aakish asked.

"Oh yes! Breakfast is ready. I will rush", she answered and banged the door quickly to avoid the conversation.

She got her reports by afternoon and found few ranges out of place. Worried about the results, she called the clinic. The slots were all full however the receptionist advised her to walk-in without an appointment.

This time Anin was more confident, and the receptionist was kind enough to allow her to see the doctor at once. Doctor checked her reports and confirmed that its Hypothyroidism, however assured her that it can be controlled with medicines after which the pregnancy can be planned. The doctor prescribed her a tablet for three months in empty stomach, first thing in the morning. She also added that there are no complications as per the pre-health checks so there is nothing to worry.

Aakish felt Anin's restlessness and tried asking her as well but never got an appropriate answer. He was not aware of the happenings as she kept it all secret. Sad for no reason, one day she finally spoke to Aakish about her worries. As expected, he was all caring and showering his love the next moment.

"Thyroid is no big deal and who is worried about having a baby anyways. Three months will pass with the blink of an eye and we can go together for the checks", he said.

I guess that was all she needed.

Aakish's words have always been musical to Anin's ears. She too realized that her fears are taking over at times. She started planning her day and felt better with her organized schedule. None of them were in hurry for the baby but with each passing day, she was getting closer to her plans of having the sweet bunch of happiness in her arms. Even though independent, women enjoy the special attention of husband accompanying them for their routine checks during early motherhood days. Going together for routine checks and tests somehow rejuvenates the bonding between the couple. The same was with Aakish and Anin.

Three months passed; it was time for the retest and Aakish accompanying her to the clinic was a real sweet gesture. After collecting the reports, they went to the doctor for consultation and it was all good!

# The New November

It was November and Aakish wanted a long vacation. In the hope to add more happy memories, they booked their tickets and were all set for the November end party. December end parties are crowded, so the first half of December was Anin's choice for a cool and calm vacation.

It was meant to be a secret, but I was sure to know it from her. Anin is not an extrovert, however, when she starts talking, she just does not stop, and I do not interrupt. Who would not want to hear her anyways!

Christmas morning was over-whelming, and she shared her experiences with all.

Off she goes:

"The perception, the fear, the feeling of getting lost dispels once you dive into it. Priorities change for good. Losing yourself for the new beginning is not easy; bouncing back with the time bravely is the key."

We had a wonderful vacation; soothing beaches, white sand, the loud waves, and the calm atmosphere was enchanting. It took our breath away! We were near the Pacific Ocean and the cabbie was from India. On the way, he showed us some wonderful places and was all smiling. We started with puran-polis (a sweet delicacy from Maharashtra) of India and by the time we reached our resort, we were talking about the sea food destinations!

It was all exciting. Our resort was beautiful, and we were delighted with the welcome drink. Coconut cooler with mint, my all-time favorite and Aakish's mango punch was a great start. The person at the reception offered us the room keys wrapped in a beautiful cloth envelope. The room was well organized, spacious, and most importantly the view of the sea was fulfilling. We were in a different world and it was no less than heaven. The resort hosted a weeklong food festival starting with Italian dishes, Persian cuisine, Indian delicacies, Lebanese food and more. Our plan for the evenings were fixed; we used to get ready by seven, enjoy the wonderful starry night and relish the delicacies. Guys at the hotel reception were very prompt and friendly. We used to get the invitation cards in the morning with all the details about the evening event. Evening musical concerts used to start by eight. The best part of the musical evenings was the location, the beach side stage for the artists and small open huts with flowers and candles for the guests. It was lovely. We used to spend the first half of the night at the beach. Sitting quietly in the love seat and counting the never-ending waves was one the things that I can never forget.

I have spent hours staring at the sky, watching the stars twinkle, glow, and fade. Watching the clouds play with the moon was always dear to me, but I never got the opportunity to watch it for hours. For people, travelling is common. For me, it is not. Am not a frequent traveler. It was special. I wanted to live every bit of it. We were in a different world; our phones were not reachable. Offices and meetings got buried in the sand and we were on top of it. We were lost in the beauty of heavens. Our routine was to sleep late yet wake up early, drive towards the east and reach before the sunrise to capture the rising sun, back to the hotel for the exhaustive breakfast buffet and then rest for a while.

We were nearing the end of our vacation, so we decided to relax at the hotel for the last few days. Lazy days: we spent time at the beach enjoying the cool and fresh drinks therein. Watching people at the fabulous sandy beach was one of our favorites. We dreamt of owning a piece of land over there and launching a beach side restaurant too!

Oh! the thoughts and imaginations were endless, but we knew that it would be the same office, same people, our friends, and the daily schedule of rush. We sat together holding hands for hours; we promised each other that we will repeat every bit of it with the little one, and with the little joy, we will go places. We then packed our bags with a smile and boarded the plane.

Paused…

# The Secret Disclosure

Anin got severe back pain, the following year. She knew that it had nothing to do with the pregnancy. The struggle went on for a couple of months. A temporary relaxation technique was finalized by her physiotherapist considering her pregnancy plans. The doctor also reminded her that the mind plays a greater role in our wellbeing and could ferry us across the seas.

Change of lifestyle and stress levels are crucial when we plan for pregnancy. Anin was thoughtful about her pregnancy plan and took all preventive measures. She tried relaxing as much as possible; ensured back support and was regular with her physiotherapist. Slowly she regained her normal routine. Thyroid was in control and so was the back pain.

I request all the women to discuss your health-related issues with your gynecologist before planning the pregnancy. This is to ensure that the pregnancy phases are convenient for you and your family.

In the month of march, Anin celebrated her pregnancy and was super excited to share the news with her love, Aakish. It was early in the morning and she went through all the blogs over the internet to confirm about the pregnancy tests at home. To reconfirm, she opted for the lab test. The gentleman at lab was supposed to send her the reports in three hours and Anin eagerly waited. It was positive! She was pregnant and it was incredibly special. A special feeling, a special day, a special moment. Everything was special. She went home, decorated her cozy corner, and prepared Aakish's favorite, the Turkish delight. It was wonderful. I have never seen her as happy as she was that day.

Aakish was also surprised with all the arrangements. It was not the usual her.

"What's so special today? Did you get promoted by any chance?" Aakish asked.

Yes, I got promoted and you as well!

"What?" he asked again.

She showed him the mail from the hospital. He read it and smiled. The smile that Anin would never ever forget. He kissed her. Soft music, dance, and dinner. Love was in the air, once again. It was their big day, the day of happiness, smiles and elated love.

The love and bonding which the pregnancy news brings with it, is eternal!

# Experiences of a New Mom

# New Happiness and Hidden Secrets of First Trimester

Anin was in her world of joy and adaptability and I was away for more than two years. I missed our pumpkins birthday but was not deprived of the feelings and the happenings around.

When we met, I asked Anin about her experiences. That is when we decided to publish a book about her journey towards motherhood, the girly thoughts, the fear, the happiness, newborn care, new mom's trouble, and a new world of discovery.

Anin wanted me to publish even the 'small and silly', not just the 'sour and sweet' things. She wanted to impart her experiences in her own words so that its shared "as-is" with the world around.

So here goes the mom's story in her own words:

Ovulation cycle varies from person to person. For me, it was sixteen (16) days, and I spent time in making sure that I know the fertile window correctly while planning my pregnancy. My doctor provided me with prenatal vitamins, and I feel that helped me a lot so ensure that you talk to your doctor about your pregnancy plans. There are few restrictions towards consumption of medicines during pregnancy so before consuming any of the medicines, even if it is for common cold, it is advisable to speak to the doctor unless you know it for sure. I was hesitant to call my doctor for silly things at first but later I developed the habit of texting her and reconfirming everything; am glad to say that she was very cooperative. Girls! call your doctor and text her as many times as you want in a day. You are solely responsible for the wellbeing of the little creature in you and there is no room for shyness.

I have heard my friends saying that men do not have any major role during the pregnancy period, however, I feel otherwise as the onus starts the day you plan your pregnancy. Proper diet, medication intake, smoking and stress level does affect the hormones. It is vital in pregnancy planning and men are required to keep a check on it. First trimester is more of a roller coaster ride and taking care of yourself is important. If the initial days come with an additional emotional support from the partner, it is always easy for the new mother-to-be to fine-tune the 'new her'.

First pregnancy is like "first love". Sun no longer imparts heat rather smiles back at you early in the morning and gives you the perfect warmth. Extraordinary and spiritual. I am not a fairy tales type personality; the responsibility was huge for me and cute at the same time. I was not yet a mom but was already daydreaming. I was cautiously walking, carefully bending, and was slowly picking up the newspaper thrown outside the door. I was such a fool to think that me doing the usual things in normal pace would hurt the baby. Not that I was not aware of the security the womb provides, but it was my way of dealing with it.

Aakish used to wake up early and ask me about my wellbeing every day. He used to drop me at office, often reminding me of not sharing the news with anyone for initial few days. Even I was of the same opinion and so I decided to keep this little secret with me. Thankfully, all was good, but I feel that we should have shared the news with all. Informing people around you about your health conditions make your life easier and secure, especially when you spend all your day with them.

I started reading about pregnancy facts and myths. My mobile notifications were showering both useful and useless knowledge. I went through all the related blogs, positiveness and even the fear part of it because I knew that fear was hidden somewhere, within me. Knowledge is great but thinking about the associated fear is not necessary.

The first new thing that I learned in my trimester was the calculation of the nine months period. I was unaware that the pregnancy counts of trimester starts from the last menstrual cycle date. My doctor maintained two hundred and eighty (280) days for my pregnancy record book, that is forty (40) weeks. Oh yes, I had a medical book for tracking the nine months of journey and I still treasure it!

My concern was the morning sickness. I was not able to escape it for first few weeks but then it disappeared. Bodily appearance does not change much during initial months and weight gain is also seen as less to nil, though there are few exceptions. I heard about pregnancy glow, lower abdominal pain, leg cramps and more but never had any of these in extreme. I had leg cramps all through my pregnancy. Every pregnancy is different so my experience might be different, however, the precautions and care needed would mostly be the same. During the first trimester, regular medications as per doctor's advice, proper diet and resting can cover it all. My doctor asked me to avoid few fruits like papaya etc. throughout my pregnancy and have everything else in moderation. I followed that and never had any issues with the diet. I continued with medications like vitamins and folic acid for few weeks but then my medications changed as per the reports. Its recommended to have an early scan within six to seven (6-7) weeks to ensure that everything is perfect and there are no health concerns. Science has reached beyond our imaginations and I understood that almost everything can be cured or controlled if detected early so there is no need to fear.

My doctor recommended few blood checks, noted down my medical history and allergies in the pregnancy record book during my first trimester. She also gave me a probable due date as per the scan results. At this time, a physical examination might happen. I had it, but there is nothing to get scared of. It does not hurt. Trusting the doctor and having confidence is the key to it. Trust yourself, be bold and you will never fail. I enjoyed my first scan; the day I saw our sweet little joy moving inside me. I heard baby's heartbeat. The moving images were making it difficult for me to identify the baby. It was not noticeably clear; the sonographer helped me identify the face, hands, and legs. Aakish loved our first scan with the baby.

First trimester is important as it is the time of change, acceptance, and caution. Morning sickness is not time bound; it can happen any time during the day. I was able to manage my office with it as it was not that bad for me. Hormonal changes, irritability, being unsettled are all part of pregnancy so you cannot get away with it but keeping yourself busy, walking and working helps in maintaining the physical and mental balance.

Its normal to think about your future, altered lifestyle and more. You will have plenty of time to do that so let the first trimester be the time to stay calm and stress free.

Life will throw challenges and we will sail through it. We have done it in the past. We will survive it in future as well, and this time for a sweet reason. Understand well that knowledge is strength but if it worries you, then verify the fact with your doctor. It is good to know about your baby's development each week as that will help you gain confidence and will keep you updated.

You may subscribe to any of the trusted magazines, or a group of experienced moms to feel better. Remember, whatever you plan to do, be it a diet change or yoga, always consult your doctor before initiating it. Even hospital these days offer yoga classes and meditation sessions. One common advice that I got from all was to stop the tea and coffee during the pregnancy, but my doctor never asked me to stop them completely. She allowed me to have it once a day based on my preferences though I stopped taking it eventually. You may talk to your doctor if you have concerns with it. Communicating with your partner and the doctor is the best way to keep yourself stress free. I got additional help for my household chores and that way got some extra fresh air to just sit and do nothing.

I was not showered with advices, however, I have heard from friends about the overdoses of advices that pour in, so breathe.

During pregnancy, it is good to talk openly about your disagreements and issues, at least with your partner. Advices from elders are always beneficial but check the facts rather than just going along with the myths. Anxiety and restlessness are common during pregnancy. Talking to trusted people, ideally the good thoughts, and engagement in no risk activities like making a salad can do wonders to your hormones. Watching a movie or reading books can also be a weekend makeover for people who usually stay busy.

# The Second Trimester Fun

Most of the women claim that second trimester is fun and the easiest. Morning sickness and fatigue goes off for expecting women and they start feeling more energetic. For me, even the mood swings got over. I was not ready to disclose anything at office but Aakish requested me to share the good news with all. As said earlier, we should let our colleagues know about our health conditions as early as possible, especially during the pregnancy, as they stay with us all day and in case of emergency, it would be our colleagues who will take care of us. We often think that disclosing the pregnancy related news would decrease our opportunities, however, three or nine months does not make much difference with respect to the work. When it is about the baby, everything else is secondary. It is good to disclose the pregnancy early so that people around you start caring for you.

Clear skies and gentle sun. My office road is naturally beautiful with wildflowers and jasmines; however, the flowers were merrier that day. Aakish dropped me at Gate number two (called S2); I was trying to walk as slow as I can. I was nervous and shy, smiled at everyone along the way, the gardener, the house keeping lady and the security guards. I used to do that earlier as well but this time it was different. I was not sure if I would be able to continue my job in future and was a bit emotional as well.

After our weekly meeting, I pushed my chair back. Our group lead was busy with her work. She was a hardworking lady, always wore those long earrings and perfect nail paints. She was not one of those floor favorites but was known for her direct speech. I liked her for what she truly was. We used to hang out at tea. I was not sure if I could go alone with her for the tea break, so I requested her for a two-minute discussion and shared the big news. She heard it with a big smile and congratulated me. She told me that being a lead, I have a lot of dependency on the project and so she will get me a backup soon. That was it. It was a quick one and not difficult. We then went on a tea break and continued the discussion as usual. I was not a person who gives up, so neither my late-night work stopped, nor did I stop taking additional tasks. The project manager at office got me a backup so that I can take things lightly, but I was in the flow and continued doing things on my own. Then one day our group lead called me for a meeting and made me realize that I could be in trouble, and that the project will suffer as well. It took me a while to comprehend but I backed off and soon started delegating my work.

I dedicated my evenings for my pregnancy checklists and started reading about it. I was feeling better. Periodic leg cramps were there but I was getting used to it. Eating right was the key. I ate loads of veggies and fruits. Second trimester was the right time to start my pregnancy walks, doing soft exercises, and joining the yoga session at doctor's advice. Second trimester was fun, and it bestowed me with the "me time". There were a lot of changes like heaviness in my breasts by the fifth month, skin stretches and more. I have heard that some women experience the heaviness in the first trimester itself, but as said earlier, every pregnancy is different.

I had a lengthy second trimester scan. Doctor explained us everything in detail and showed us the small arms, eyes (was difficult to distinguish though), the heartbeat and all other body parts. Aakish was excited about it. The baby was folding his hand again and the doctor told us that he is kind of doing the "namaste pose". We enjoyed it. It was fun, exciting, and loving all together.

Development was good and no birth defects were detected, so it ended well and this time we got some additional pictures as well.

It was not long that I entered my seventh month of pregnancy. I opted for the pregnancy package at the hospital. There were lot of options like semi-private rooms, private ones, luxury, etc. Aakish made the choice for the room and took some additional options as well for our comfort.

A hospital near to the house is a bliss and if you have the option to start your checks early at the same place, it is always good. I was lucky that my doctor was associated with the women's hospital near to our place and so I opted for it without any second thought.

It was a good decision for both of us considering we had less help and more of responsibilities.

# The Busy Third Trimester

My doctor prescribed a separate dose specifically for two weeks based on my scan results and asked me to take complete rest. I was already in my happiest phases, so I applied for my sick leaves based on my reports. It was one of the best decisions that I ever took. Though I missed working with some of my good friends at office, the leave was a necessity based on my health conditions.

Am proud of them who plan to continue the work till the last day of pregnancy and its great, but I always wanted it the other way. I started shopping online and completed my checklists for the post-pregnancy needs. I started spending time in our butterfly garden; it was wonderful. At times it was boring and irritating as well, but that's part of hormonal changes. Backache was hitting me often during my third trimester and the leg cramps kept me awake all night. It was difficult to walk with a big sized body; I was consistently gaining weight. My friends advised me to take short walks, however, I was too lazy for that. I stopped going to my yoga classes as well. Not walking enough was the biggest of mistakes I made during my last trimester. The only good activity that I religiously followed was the dinner preparation and that helped me stay active late evenings.

Frequency of appointments with the health care professionals increase at the later stages which is good for the overall development checks. Baby kick count increases with the growth. For me, the baby was active most of the time, especially at nights.

Stretching of skin is irritating but it is sure to happen, moisturizing being the only way out unless it is bad, and you plan for a doctor's visit. Headache, swelling of hands and feet, etc. were also part of my pregnancy journey. Lower back pain was common for me; however, I was dealing with the issues and was getting over it.

If there is anything that you feel is not normal, you must see the health care professionals.

The third trimester scan was interesting. We were able to identify the baby's arms, legs, and head without any help from the sonographer. Even the movements were clear. The positioning of the baby was not appropriate as per the scan and we knew that it could lead us to a major delivery procedural change. Our doctor requested us to have patience. Considering that the baby changes its position until the last minute, we were calm.

I felt that the periodic scans encourage bonding with the baby apart from its medical mandates. Forty-five minutes of lovely exploration was something we used to wait for! We were able to talk endlessly about the baby after the scan. For me, the baby would be sleeping during my scans and eating a piece of chocolate would turn the little one super active. It was hilarious!

It is good to have the same doctor throughout the pregnancy unless there is a good reason for the change. First trimester would be ideal for the shift but if you have no options, do not worry about it; doctors will anyways take care of it. They are all experts.

Thankfully, mine was a normal delivery, however, I did ask my doctor about epidurals during my last trimester. I wanted to know if it really helps in reducing the delivery pains. Doctor answered in affirmative and told me that it does help to an extent but there are other factors to be considered as well. She told me that the epidural experts are assigned to perform the procedures, but the gynecologists will be there for the delivery. In normal conditions, they prefer the natural process. There will obviously be factors like positioning, delays, baby's heart rate, etc. which will be considered before administering the same if the lady opts for the epidurals. The epidural experts and health care professionals will always be the right people to guide you. I did speak to some of the hospital staffs. Talking to people who get involve in the actual process was my way of gaining confidence. I did ask my doctor about my periodic leg cramps and itching. She said its normal to have them based on my condition, however, if its unbearable then we will have to take care of it with few additional tests. Mine was not that bad so I did not go for any tests.

Eighth and ninth month gives you the feeling of the lovely bundle of joy growing inside. I was not able to sleep on my tummy for a year, so I had only two options; either sleep on my sides which was never comfortable for me or sit with a support on the back. Counting the kicks was one of the few tasks during the final months of pregnancy. Kicks usually do not hurt but keep reminding you of the super active baby. It was a new experience for me.

Sharing cupcakes during the baby shower and the lovely wrist corsage bracelet will enhance your day for sure. Trust me! Celebrating baby shower with friends helps in reducing the anxiety. My baby shower gifts were loaded with love; newborn diapers, spa packages and more but for me, the most exciting gift was the wish that the guests whispered in my ears as per our tradition.

We often say that love is fascinating and amazing when shared but being the foundation of love is a wonderful feeling. What if your soul feels the same and your universe starts revolving around it? That is what happens in the third trimester. It is all in the mind, but social interaction plays an integral part. It is the time to think positive. Eighth month was roses, beautiful butterfly gardens, pool sit outs, matinee shows at home and more, however, birth planning was also on my list of activities. Whether you want a normal delivery, C-section or epidural, it is good to read, think, discuss with your partner, and finalize. Of course, we cannot control the last-minute changes as per doctor's advice but if things go as per the plan, moms will have additional confidence.

# Checklists for the Big Day

Birth planning also includes the hospital baggage checklist.

**Must have for mommies:**

Hospital slippers

Free size dress with nursing zippers

Few pairs of socks

Nursing brassiere and Maternity pads

Toiletries like perfumes, towels, hairbrush, toothbrush, hair clips, lip balm and more

Going back home outfit

Camera to capture the first moments with the precious one.

**First day needs for the small bundle of joy:**

Muslin cloths and baby wraps

Baby blankets and cozy envelopes for the little ones

Soft cotton newborn wear

Pair of booties for the new baby

Nappies for the loved one

You can add more to it but try to keep it as per the need to ensure that your baggage is friendly.

# Impatient World

# Restlessness All Around

Although I was in my own sweet thoughts, ninth month taught me about the society and the impatient world that exists in full swing. Good wishes and gifts, I was treated like a celebrity during the last phase of pregnancy. Neighbors started inviting me for lunch. I realized that the ritual of feeding pregnant ladies is still considered auspicious and is celebrated in India with all enthusiasm.

With the impatient people around, I also lost my patience at times. I wanted all of it to get over at once, but it does not happen that way. All phases are equally important for the growth of the baby. Walking and standing was getting difficult, waist level discomfort was adding to my frustrations and I lost my sleep and calmness. Part of it was excitement, part of it was fear but mostly it was my mind who was impatient.

Aakish used to impart long narrations on relaxation benefits but am not sure if I remember all of those for others to benefit from. Those days even my dreams were more of a reflection of my conscious and subconscious mind, inclined towards the baby and birthing techniques.

Butterfly gardens no longer fascinated me and all I wanted to do was to gaze at the calendar, count the number of days left for the big day and pack my bags. I was lazy and was not moving much so Aakish used to kept me on my toes whenever possible.

Finding the right name for the baby was the best thing to do and the game of "funny names" with your friends and well-wishers, a great stress buster. Spend time on the name as your baby will be known by it. Translate the name to ensure that you know the meaning of it in other languages as well if that bothers you. It is always difficult to find a perfect name for the precious one unless you already have your favorites ready, so enjoy your days with the "name-search" for the little one.

I would advise all to get as much sleep as possible and indulge in less stressful activities at home. Get a little me-time, a pampering pedicure, watch movies and have peaceful moments with your husband and loved ones. Once the baby free days end, load of chores follows.

# Bliss

Christmas was getting closer, and I was excited. My due date was on 25th of December and it was making me more restless. I entered my last week of pregnancy; Aakish applied for his leaves and handled my fears and frustrations boldly and calmly, as always. Until Wednesday of the final week, it was all good; we both gave fear a back seat and enjoyed our candle night dinners, continental breakfasts and more. Thursday morning was for real and we were tensed. I started checking my arrangements. It was a get-set-go for us, however, we thought of having our lunch and rest for a while before proceeding. I was not hungry, I was a little excited, a little scared and a little restless. We planned a grand welcome for the little one with flowers, cakes, toys and more.

Few things that bothered me before getting ready was personal and hence I called the hospital. I requested the receptionist to transfer me to the nursing department of delivery and the head of nursing gladly answered all my queries. The turmoil of thoughts that a women might have at the hour may vary, but it is necessary to unfold your heart and inquire, because the mission ahead would need a lot of patience and confidence.

I was secretly preparing myself for the future. Our hospital was few miles away and in no time we were there. We witnessed a car getting decorated with blue balloons at the parking and were able to relate the blessings that the new mother carried in her arms. I was not panicking but was nervous; we went to the second-floor maternity house; the room was all set for us. It was spacious and smelled like lemon, was artfully arranged.

My first conversation with the nursing staff was full of assurance.

"What is you name?", I asked her.

"Seena", she replied.

She was all smiling, and I was nervous.

"Relax and have a nice stay here. We will arrange the food for you so please ensure that you eat only the food provided by us and nothing else from outside. We will start the routine check in an hour", she said.

"What checks?", I asked her anxiously.

"The procedurals. Don't worry about it", she replied.

After an hour, the duty doctor entered my room. She smiled and got my blood pressure checked. Her words were polite but scary. I started practicing the breathing techniques that I learnt during my early pregnancy yoga sessions. I was aware of the slow dancing techniques that help stay calm before the delivery but instead of trying them, I gave myself a sheepish giggle. I feared the scary cesarean stories about "late recoveries", "the struggles to lose weight", etc. Little did I knew that there is nothing normal about the normal delivery that I was hoping for. Epidural was my only hope and I rested on it. Aakish was tensed with my nonstop worries and fears, he tried his best to keep me relaxed. Amidst all this, I was reminding him to enquire about the pediatrician. The hospital staff however asked us not to worry as the initial screening and checks of the newborn was included in our package.

Some parents who opted for cord blood banking had to perform some additional formalities; we did not opt for it for some personal reasons. It is said that the umbilical cord is the richest source of stem cells and it can treat several medical conditions in future. The details on these are usually explained during the scheduled hospital visits so if you are unsure, it is good to speak to your doctor early.

My contractions were getting intense. Procedures were endless: cleansing the stomach, pre-medications, preparing your body for the next steps, etc. Good thing was that the nurses were friendly, caring and were explaining the procedures well. It was midnight and I was sleepy but who can sleep peacefully with contractions anyways! Giving birth is difficult however, trusting the doctors and nurses at the hospital is important and it adds to the confidence.

I was asked not to take any more food. Pre procedures were smooth and exactly at seven in the morning, they took me to the labor room. The equipment's were scary, but I maintained my calmness. I saw my doctor approaching me with some boxes and gauzes.

My conversation with the health care professionals was bold and confident, as always, but I was scared, very scared.

Good morning, the doctor said.

All I would need from you is trust and confidence. I will take care of the rest. I will be back in sometime; she added.

The delivery nurse came and introduced herself. Sister Sarita was young and confident.

"Will it be very painful? How long will it take?", I asked.

"We will give painkillers as per the procedure so don't worry about it. I will help you with your delivery, so relax and stay calm. Your husband is also allowed in the labor room during the birthing procedure, you will feel better with Mr. Aakish being here", she explained calmly.

"We will start with the epidural. This will give you some relief. Mr. Abraham is our epidural expert, and he will be here in a moment ", said Sarita.

Dr. Abraham was a senior doctor, it was not a surprise for me. He introduced himself and asked me to move around the room and relax before starting with the epidural.

"Will it hurt?", I asked the doctor.

"No, not at all. It will save you from the pain and it just feels like an ant bite", he answered.

Aakish was asked to go out during the epidural procedure. Today epidural has become one of the popular form of medication-based pain relief. It is always good to read and discuss about pain relief options available before pregnancy. My doctor explained me that epidural is more of a regional anesthesia that blocks the nerve impulses from lower spinal segments so that the sensation from the lower half of the body is decreased. The relief depends on the type of epidural procedures chosen by you. There are few downsides of this as well, so doctors are always the best guides.

I was feeling the pain even after the epidural procedures, but it was relatively low. The contractions kept getting stronger and I requested the doctor to infuse more pain relief if that was possible. In my case the labor did prolong. Usually, its active labor and then few hours until the childbirth but mine went on and on and on. Finally, with forceps delivery, it took seven hours for my bundle of joy to arrive. Nurse Sarita managed to push the baby down and made it happen; I gave up too early. All I remember was getting a glance of the baby's hands and then few hours of semiconsciousness. I heard doctor's claiming that it is a boy but could not stay awake to see the baby. Aakish took care of him and followed him to the Newborn Intensive Care Unit. Newborns are secured in an appropriate environment at the intensive care for few hours. The baby was the first thing I asked for after gaining my consciousness. The nurses then took me back to my room, got me cleaned, padded, and made me comfortable. I cannot thank them enough for helping me. They went an extra mile to make me comfortable. Aakish was on and off. Few minutes with me and few minutes with the baby at the intensive care. He was tired, had red eyes and all he wanted was to get the baby quickly next to me. It was around 3:45PM. Epidural affect kept me drowsy, and I was sleeping every now and then. Just then my baby arrived, and I saw him for the first time. Cute bundle of joy and smiles; it was the most wonderful feeling of this world! I do not think anyone till date has words to express this special feeling; I would leave it for the would-be-moms to experience.

The nurse wanted me to try breastfeeding, but I was not comfortable, so she gave him the infant formula or the baby milk. Aakish took the little one in his arms, he was incredibly happy and hungry at the same time. I requested him to take his food while I keep an eye on the little one. Aakish went upstairs and got his food packed. The nutritionist, lactation consultant, exercise manuals and other details kept me awake all day. I was hardly listening to any of those guys, but they did their job well. Aakish was taking care of the baby meanwhile. Men do not experience the physical trauma or the hormonal changes that an women do however, they need a bagful of patience to survive in the see-saw environment of an expecting women; It only adds up as the little one arrives. Feeding and baby poops continued. With a little tummy, his intake was small and therefore he was capable enough to keep his father awake for one more night!

Next day, I was able to walk with support from others. I was also able to take care of the baby but not for long. My baby was not able to latch so infant formula was the only hope; however, the nurses encouraged me to keep trying every two hours. The nutritionist handed me over the diet chart and asked me to follow it for at least fifteen days for faster recovery. I slept again for few hours. Aakish was very tired. It was obvious. I then took the baby in my arms. Though Aakish tried sleeping, his sleep was getting disturbed every ten minutes either because of the gift hampers from the hospital or the decoration of the door with blue balloons. I was excited to go back home with the little one; I was weak and had little patience to execute our idea of celebration, but a quick photo session with the little one was a wonderful start. Aakish managed to get the flowers for the entrance, and we were excited about the first day at home.

# Loosing Selfhood

# Postpartum/Postnatal Issues

Arriving at home and welcoming the new member in our own special way was overwhelming. By the time we settled down, the little one was awake and screaming. Without the luxury of nurses and domestic help at home; it was tough.

The pediatrician at the hospital who administered the preliminary vaccination for the baby, told me to ensure that the baby feeds on breast and not to bank on the infant formula, however, it was not an easy task. With consistent effort and the help of lactation consultants, I was slowly able to breastfeed him. Positioning the baby right and ensuring that the nose is not getting pressed is important to note while breastfeeding. Co-sleeping with the baby helps; however, we need to ensure that the milk does not leak and flow into baby's ears while feeding. We must be vigilant all day and all night, so additional help during initial days is a must. Burping is crucial for the baby. The nurse usually explains the procedure of patting the back for the burp. If not, you can always ask.

I was in the recovery stage and my baby was getting used to the new environment. Body pain was bad for me. Post-delivery massage helped me, but it was a personal choice; It is advisable to talk to your doctor about the same as the delivery procedures and their impact on the body differs. Similarly, the baby bath and massage start date (if willing to) must be discussed with the doctor. In our culture, baby massage was important however some doctors voted against it. Initially I felt that the breastfeeding was not enough as the baby was crying hard and loud often, but later my gynecologist prescribed me an ayurvedic medicine that is usually taken by the new mom's and it helped!

Consoling the baby, waking up every fifteen minutes at night was a ritual then. There were issues but I got over it. First week was difficult and first night with the baby was impossible. He cried all night. It took time for him to adapt. After a week, I felt that we were all adapting to the environment. My patience was always on a roller coaster ride. I lost myself while taking care of the newborn. I used to forget my medicines at times. Once I forgot brushing my teeth and was reminded of it only when the food tasted weird. I forgot my dinner, the boiling milk, the running tap and more. Aakish was out of my sight most of the times and all my focus was on the baby. Adhering to his needs and taking care of him was primary and rest all was secondary for me. His routines were mine and his changing habits were adapted by me as well. It is easy to write about him because there is so much to it, however, few things are better felt than spoken. Do spend some time with the little one after the feed. The baby usually smiles at that time and it comes for a fraction of second but holds the power to leave you smiling for hours, amidst all the pain.

In early weeks, Aakish's swaddling the baby and helping with the sleep time routine was bestowing me with few additional minutes, however, the primary responsibility was always mine. I was getting used to the sleepless nights, breastfeeding and the baby was enjoying his cuddle time. Keeping him calm, relaxed, happy, with proper food and burps was keeping me busy. My responsibilities and duties got confined within the house. I was not going for the park walk as I wanted the baby to stay indoors for initial few weeks. Aakish did extend his leaves, however, I was against it. With no alternatives, my cook was my baby's nanny for three-to-four hours a day. We hired a lady for the baby massage and bath, she was a professional and my baby started loving his bath and play time.

I never came across any scientific evidence of baby catching the cold from breastmilk, but few people advised me to stop taking cold and chilled food, ice-creams etc. It was not making sense to me; however, I knew that moms could pass the cold viruses with sneeze or breath, so I took care of myself and tried avoiding the chilled foods, especially the soft drinks and ice-creams for a while. After a month of never-ending nappies, feeding, humming; I was frustrated. Getting up at night was a routine with no exception. It would either be a growth spurt or a pain in the stomach for him and I would stay awake all night. I felt as if I was paving my way towards depression but was capable enough to bounce back with positive thoughts.

All the ladies out there must know that it is just a phase and it will pass. I was extremely cautious about the baby and ensured that I never take out my frustrations on him. After a month I started going out with the baby. Trust me, the walk not just helps the baby interact with the environment but also gives the new mom a breath full of energy and enthusiasm.

I was aware of my mood swings and started making efforts to get away with it. I used to pump and store extra milk so that Aakish can feed the baby as well. Eventually I got a full-time nanny for the baby and started setting expectations with her however, my baby was not getting well with her. She was a well-trained babysitter, but I feel it is more of the willingness and love that matters when you deal with the baby along with the training. Anyways, we survived!

# Learnings from the Sleepless Nights

1: Trusting yourself and keeping the confidence high can help outsmart all odds.

2: A tired mind and body can hurt, and both stay together post pregnancy. Keep calm, its crucial for your wellbeing.

3: House help during initial days is a must. This is necessary because nurses do not follow you home.

4: Listen to doctor's advice on tips to overcome the initial period of uncertainty. Meet lactation consultant at hospital with positive and attentive mindset to ensure that you know the breastfeeding guidelines and positioning. This will save you from backaches and stress.

5: Painkillers prescribed by your gynecologist work like the life savers on initial days but stick to your doctor's prescription. If you feel the need to take more, talk to your doctor first.

6: Newborns are delicate so we must be careful and attentive towards them even at the toughest of hours.

7: Partners can help with the baby's sleep routine and that is no less than the pain killer.

8: Its ok to get frustrated, nervous and feel depressed at times however, its necessary that we bounce back soon with confidence and strength; after all its just a phase and it would change for good.

9: Talking to people and joining trusted groups for a discussion or sharing of thoughts is good for new moms. College group or your old school talks work no less than peacemakers.

10: Sleep when the baby sleeps. Its ok to sleep and sleep and sleep if needed; the world can wait.

# Beating Anxiety and Depression

Morning air, evening walks, music at times, and joining new moms' group helps in fighting the depression out. Do these things even if you feel that you do not need to. There is nothing better than talking to the family members and friends. Ordering the grocery can also be a stressbuster at times. Opting for home spa services or just a pedicure feels great so try them as well!

If there is anyone you can talk to, you must. Take the opportunity to laugh your heart out even at the silliest of jokes and keep the troubling elements/thoughts away.

Watch stand-up comedy shows, hilarious movies or anything that interests you, even though in bits and pieces. It can work wonders. When evening unfolds, the babies usually get irritated, so an afternoon nap is mandatory. Just lie down and relax in the afternoon even if you do not get a good sleep. Instead of getting irritated, enjoy the positivity of this phase. There will be sleepless nights at length for sure.

Teething is one of the crucial stages in baby's life. My baby got fever during the third month when he got his first teeth. Loose motions did not accompany him and that was a relief. I used to be on my toes all night and hardly got time to lie down. It took a weeks' time for him to get out of the irritability and sleeplessness. At times I felt low, however, I learnt patience, love, and tolerance.

When it is all good, prepare for an official weekend photoshoot with the baby and enjoy the day with the family.

Walk to the nearby supermarket if you are willing to, even if it is just a packet of milk that you would need. Always ensure that you have someone to accompany you and keep your hands free when you go out. Let the stroller carry the milk and water bottle for the baby.

Self-motivation and keeping yourself busy with the little things you love is a great practice. Gardening if you love, is one of the best things that you can work on along with the baby.

Read books or just cook an easy meal; do whatever makes you happy. Ensure that you never approve a sad pause.

# Plums and Pumpkins

# Babies' Milestones and Solids

My baby was in his seventh month and I was approaching my maternity leave completion date. Joining the workplace back was in my mind. The small hands grabbed me, and I stretched my leaves to the maximum possible days. Starting solids was my next target for the baby and we celebrated it with great enthusiasm. With only our dearest of friends, we managed a small get-together. Fortunately, the baby was also in good mood, however, following day he got loose motions. Doctor advised us to hold on for few days before starting up with solids and gave us few oral medicines to calm the baby. Changing the diapers more than fifteen times a day was not fun. When baby's stomach gets upset, it is advisable to use a cotton cloth dipped in lukewarm water instead of using the wipes at frequent intervals. I did not follow that, and the diaper rashes were evident; my baby was not in peace for two days. Slowly with the external medications, things settled down and we started with the solids again.

I feel that the three-day rule for food is a must for all babies: we should introduce one new food at a time and wait for three days before introducing another. That way it is easier for the baby to adapt and we can isolate the food allergies if any. Some babies are allergic to egg and dry fruits. Light and easily digested foods are always advised while starting with the solids. For my baby, it was "boiled and mashed apple"; one spoon per day. My baby liked it on the third day. The second food I introduced was pulses. I was conservative with the food introduction process, especially after his stomach infections. He slowly started loving it; smooth textures were his favorites as those were easy to gulp. He loved smoothies as well. Boiled raw papaya is great, but the amount of papaya should be less, else the baby gets an upset stomach.

Colic is common among babies. It is not confined to solid starters. Even newborns get colic at times, so it is important to have colic medicines handy as per the pediatrics advice. Touching the baby's stomach gently can help identify colic to some extent. The baby with colic sleeps well in arms but wakes up as soon as you put him in the bed, however, this can be a sign for baby's idea of coziness as well. It takes a lot of patience and understanding to identify the cries and the associated needs.

The little explorers get more curious once they reach the sixth and seventh month. They start learning about the environment. They love to explore; slowly they start moving (crawling, getting up with support and then the first independent step follows). As they reach these milestones, they need more attention and keep their moms and caretakers busy.

Keeping track of the vaccination is important; discussions with the pediatrician about the new developments and concerns is vital.

In between sixth and seventh month, my baby started showing excitement and happiness. He was making babbling sounds, getting curious about partially hidden objects, was responding to his name and more. He was fascinated with his mirror images. He started sitting without any support in the seventh month, but it is normal for babies to reach a little early or take some more time to achieve these milestones. Playing with the baby and a little encouragement with movements helps the baby achieve the milestones with less effort.

Within nine months, I was playing a detective. The baby started taking objects to his mouth and I used to watch him all day, nonstop. He played tricks and I enjoyed them too. He was loving the sound of the falling objects and was trying his hands with everything that was reachable. He started understanding the word 'no', but he was not obedient towards it.

Some babies start displaying the separation anxiety by eighth or ninth month as well but if the routine is followed, they adapt soon.

The tenth, eleventh and twelfth month passed with a blink of an eye. Lot of things came together. The baby started communicating with waves and sounds and with pointers, however, the curious one managed to keep us alert and active all the while. He not just showed his affection but also started displaying his preferences. He sounded super cute while imitating our words and at the same time ensured that he turns the house topsy-turvy. Shaking, banging, throwing, and dropping were his favorites and he was quickly trying to stand without support, falling multiple times. He needed a person always by his side. With all the nonstop experiments, it is good to get help rather than trying to achieve everything on your own. I learnt it the hard way.

With birthdays, comes the first step without any support. Some babies achieve it before their birthdays and some after it. Either ways, keep encouraging them to take those little steps, one at a time.

# Beating Frustrations with Awareness

1: "Babies rolling-over" is one the most common milestone that parents look for during initial months. Every child is different so if your baby is taking time to achieve this, be patient. Do not get tensed. If unsure, talk to your pediatrician. I used to give my baby ten minutes of floor time in a thick baby mat when he was three months old and was continuous putting efforts to roll over. I used to stay with the baby while he is in the mat to ensure that he is not struggling with it.

2: Follow three-day thumb rule to introduce solids. One type of food at a time. Always start with light and easily digested ones. Introduce food in very less quantity, it can be one spoon. This helps the baby adapt to the new food and parents get to isolate the ones that have the potential to cause allergies. Do not get disheartened or frustrated if the baby does not accept the solid food. Try again in the gap of two to three days and keep trying with different flavors.

3: It is common for a new mom to experience abdominal bloating regularly, causing discomfort. Soaking Carom (ajwain) in a cup of water and then filtering out the carom seeds thereby drinking only the water instead of tea or coffee, early in the morning, is a great way to get relief from the discomfort. Please ensure that you are not allergic to Carom seeds before drinking this. Carom seeds have several health benefits, and I was drinking it every morning as a replacement for my coffee.

4: Getting cold and cough during initial months is not usual for the babies but if it happens, home remedies can assure some relief. After the sixth month, I used to rub gentle mustard oil infused with garlic and carom seeds in the feet of the baby for warmness. I always ensured that my baby wears a soft socks after any external application to the feet. It is good to talk to the pediatrician in advance and get child friendly nasal drops along with the recommended doses for common cold and cough.

5: Homemade food is always preferred over the packed ones. Take some time out to read about them, especially the storage part of it, so that it can be stored for longer duration thereby making the process easy and less time consuming for the parents.

6: Talk to the pediatrician or the nurse at hospital about wax in the little ears and they will help you during your visits to the hospital for the regular checks. Do not try it on your own.

7: If the new-born baby throws fresh milk soon after the feeds, it could be a burp or the excess that has gone in. Check the situation and call your doctor. Most of pediatricians help you on call, so make use of the same.

8: Switch to a cloth diaper during the day or give few diaper-free hours to the baby.

9: Each baby is different so stop comparing and start enjoying the days.

10: Gentle massage for the baby worked wonderfully for me to get him a good afternoon nap but some people and doctors vote against it, so it is good to consult your pediatrician before deciding on it.

11: Painful vaccinations gives you and the baby a troublesome day, however, they are known to be more effective till date when compared to the painless ones. That is what I was told, however, you must speak to your pediatrician before deciding on it.

12: Washing baby toys and maintaining hygiene is important but they take a major chunk of free time and energy so plan the toys as per the days. This also helps in keeping the baby interested with the games. They lose interest with the toy they see every day, however, there will always be few favorites that they would look for.

13: Spend time with the baby. Playing, encouraging for movements, and talking to the little one help them achieve their milestones and offers them the much-needed assurance.

14: Independence; be it crawling, walking, or running, make children more active and enthusiastic. Always keep an eye on the baby.

15: Stick to the bedtime routines and never ever let it go. That is the only way you can plan your day and your activities.

# Super Confused Mom, Possessiveness, and the Way Out

Understanding the ups and downs of baby's behavior, discussions at new mommies' group, music and baby activities kept me occupied for few months. An experience different from the usual; I got engrossed in my new lifestyle. Obsession with hygiene and cleanliness killed all my time and I kept cleaning the toys and the house to ensure that my baby gets a germ-free environment until his immune system matures. My palms used to get dry and painful. Not sure if my approach was good but lot of people vouched against it and asked me not to overdo things. They thought that the baby would be more prone to diseases this way, however, I continued doing the same.

Maternity dresses all over; I was able to hide my stretch marks and the protruding postpartum belly. I was scheduling my spa appointments but was canceling them. I was convincing myself with the video streaming and live sessions of daycares but was not able to take any decision. For me, the cause of frustration was being directionless and my confused state of mind. Baby's daycare centers help enhance the baby's social and interactive skills. I always wanted him to share the space with other kids but not before the age of two.

Part of me was becoming super possessive and part of me was not able to trust that anyone else in this world is capable enough to take care of my baby, as I do. It is obvious and holds no shame. Keeping the baby-first attitude starts as soon as you conceive, so you would need time to convince yourself that the little one can stay without the mother, with proper guidance, for few hours a day. Take your time to settle down. Trust me girls, our well-wishers, family and even the reliable caregivers care for the baby as we do, so do not worry much. There are lot of options and arrangements available for working moms. Daycare's at early age ensures that the baby's routine is developed much early so whoever wants to adhere to the same, must explore the options.

I was not able do it, so I thought of quitting the job for few years and join back after the baby is matured enough to talk and express his feelings. It was my personal choice but not the only option for the new moms. Managing work and the baby together must be explored before taking any decisions.

I have never seen a mom regretting about anything that she has done for the baby, so I spoke to Aakish about my plans. Aakish also voted with me and we were all smiling. It was crystal clear that our decision for the baby was right. I resigned, returned my official id's thereby getting a good settlement with the final goodbye to the corporate. Things went well, however, I felt sad at times for leaving my job.

Quick pedicure and books were the best of my pals those days. With the arrivals of rains and cozy weather, my baby slept well. Aakish's life was easier than before with me leaving the job and the baby growing up becoming more independent each day. Understanding different phases of life with the baby was a great experience. I realized that any kind of learning is satisfactory, and no one stops you to enlighten yourself with the knowledge that you long for. I also tried my hands with gardening and failed several times, but I never gave up. I slowly learnt few gardening techniques to keep myself occupied. Morning glories made my mornings glow. Sunflowers taught me to respect the rising sun and the lovely white jasmines enabled me to breathe the freshness at night. Beautiful creepers paved their way to my windows. I was happy that my life was full of lovely creatures; my baby being the most adorable of them.

# A New Life – the Unbounded Discovery

# Special Birthday and a
# New Opportunity

Having a beautiful garden, a sparkling house, raising a child, creating a genius, or encouraging the next generation might be a part of the purpose, but I knew that it cannot be my only purpose in life. I was planning to start something of my own followed by some additional work for the unprivileged, but all those plans took the backstage as I was contributing towards the bonding, peace and comfort of the family while raising the little one.

Everybody was happy especially the baby because he was spending all his time with me, playing.

Our prince was turning one soon and we planned for a birthday bash! It was one of the biggest events of our life. I was confident with doughnuts and breads but this time it was a birthday cake. I thought of baking the first birthday cake for my baby. Oh yes! that was bold and Aakish was against it with all his will however, I was not ready to give up. I tried convincing him with all my baking skills but risking the cake with my half-earned skills was not something that he wanted.

We started choosing the invitation cards and professionals to plan the event based on our budget and the venue. I was good at event planning. Within a week's time, I was able to finalize all arrangements except a few, like the stage setup and the cake. We still had one month, and we knew that a lot of virtual meets will follow once the event organizers start with the actual work. It was a fairly good experience. I was not just spending my time with the organizers but was also baking flavored cakes at home. I was reassuring myself with my skills and was trying to implement all that I learnt, years ago. I was a baker since childhood but this time it was different; I wanted to create a masterpiece. Our event organizers requested for the sign off on cakes, but I delayed it.

It was a Sunday and I started baking a prototype. It took me six long hours and it came out perfect! Aakish loved it and we decided to bake our own cake for our son's first birthday.

On his birthday night, with ease, I baked three cakes. The idea was to have a three-layered cake with different flavors. It was winter and Igloo was the theme; It was no less than a masterpiece. Aakish helped me in the process as always. We were deprived of sleep but were not deprived of our energy levels.

Our sunshine, Arit's birthday was special for all of us. It was a busy day and Arit was surprisingly cooperative. The birthday evening flowed in and the soothing music established perfect harmony. Love, balloons, and the colorful gift wraps kept the little one busy and to our surprise he was enjoying with the people. We had games, dance and more. Everyone liked the birthday event; cake was the center of attraction. All of them were surprised to hear that the cake was baked at home and I was proudly receiving all of it! It was getting very cold outside so with heavy hearts our guests started bidding goodbye. Just then an old lady approached me and asked if I can bake a small cake for his granddaughter. She wanted a double layered cute small cake and was ready to pay in advance, but I refused the money. I told her that I will do it for her granddaughter, and she can pay me only if the birthday girl likes it. She was incredibly happy to hear that.

She was my angel!

# The Baker: End of Our Conversation

The ensuing week, I baked my second birthday cake. It was for the old lady's granddaughter. I handed over the cake to her and her granddaughters blissful bright smile said it all!

My third cake was for my neighbor. Showers of appreciations kept me elated. Soon I started getting small orders from my apartment. It was all fun and madness.

Lot of things have changed in last two years and am glad that I have evolved. Am still learning. I have a lot to learn about parenting, housekeeping, relationships, baking and more. Every day is a learning for me.

It is important that we learn to adapt and create opportunities with whatever we have now. At the same time, it is also vital that we talk to our partners and our family about our career plans, post pregnancy, to make sure that they support us in all possible ways. Women should take their decisions based on their own preferences. There should not be any place for fear or insecurity.

Am glad to have two wonderful people supporting me at home, Aakish and Arit. Aakish loves baking these days and helps me with whatever he can. My free time is all productive with additional learnings on advanced cake baking and design techniques. I have started ordering new tools. Hobby as a free time job is not much of an earning, but we are able to turn the kitchen into a lovable working space. I wish to have a cake and coffee corner someday but as of now it is just Arit that I would like to have.

Smiles…

Grace and glories; Anin's eyes were reflecting happiness and I was incredibly happy to see that.

The IT lady turned 'mom and baker' is loving her baking skills these days and when at peace, apart from talking to me she loves checking her fan page!

*I was convinced that the power of love blesses you with your day. You just have to say yes!*

Motherhood is love and there is no substitute for it. It is an experience that offers you a bundle of happiness. It is a blessing from god, a gift of a pause. A pause in life that allocates time to think, to rejoice, to love and to identify the purpose of your life, the true you!

Only we women are gifted with this extraordinary present. The procedure of taking a break and the liberty to think before joining back the world again could be a part of the plan, however, the decision to change a path or continue the one we love is completely ours. A year's break or two is not going to pull down our career so we must plan our preferences fearlessly and spend time with the little one; they deserve it!

If you plan to join back the same place where you left a while ago, brush up your skills months ahead and if possible, make yourself aware of the changes at your workplace so that when you go back, you are not surprised.

World is changing and getting more liberal while offering the same work opportunities to the working mothers, however, if you still meet someone in your way, who says or acts as if you are not capable enough to continue the job at the same pace as earlier, do smile at them.

*Astonished with my intelligence, amazed with the
stars collected,*

*Thee granted two additional points.*

*Wherefore cognizant of me being a mom, it decreased???*

*Wonder why the trust abated when I have additionally gained,*

*The knowledge, the patience, the more responsible I
have become,*

*The selflessness, the compassionate, the seriousness I
have earned,*

*For they would know the path that women have climbed, was
not the stairs that goes up and down but the leaps that only the
brave can dare!*

**Glory!**